I0436797

Six Pieces of Pie

Dealing with elderly parents as an adult child.

Ruth Marie Burke

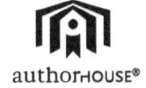

authorHOUSE®

AuthorHouse™
1663 Liberty Drive
Bloomington, IN 47403
www.authorhouse.com
Phone: 1-800-839-8640

Cover photo by Ruth Marie Burke, May, 2009

© 2009 Ruth Marie Burke. All rights reserved.

No part of this book may be reproduced, stored in a retrieval system, or transmitted by any means without the written permission of the author.

First published by AuthorHouse   7/1/2009

ISBN: 978-1-4389-9813-8 (e)
ISBN: 978-1-4389-9814-5 (sc)

Printed in the United States of America
Bloomington, Indiana

This book is printed on acid-free paper.

To:

Jason, my youngest son,
and Rich, my younger brother -

Who taught me lessons in letting go!

George and Berdina, my parents -
Who are still teaching me lessons in living!

Erik and Christopher, my two oldest sons -
Who will both have to deal with me if I live to
be an octogenarian or older!

TABLE OF CONTENTS

FORWARD

Dealing with parents who are in their late 80s and early 90s is difficult for adult children who live nearby. It is more of a challenge when situations must be dealt with from 1500 miles away! This is a depiction of one baby-boomer's dealings with geriatric maturing parents. The scope of this book provides personal stories divided into categories that depict coping with the many facets of elderly parents. Some topics include Alzheimer's disease, Parkinson's disease, organizing medications, loss of independence, and coping with the loss of a child. This is intended for information and entertainment only. Medical information pertaining to similar personal situations should be obtained during consultation with a physician.

ACKNOWLEDGEMENT

The cover photo was taken by Ruth Marie Burke. The portrayal of the lemon meringue pie is symbolic of the story woven throughout the chapters. I was able to use my mother's china dessert plate, along with my grandmother's crystal water goblet.

Six Pieces of Pie

Apple, peach, or pumpkin pie; all wonderful comfort foods when one is planning dessert for a family dinner finale. During the years when my younger brother and I were growing up, my grandmother baked marvelous German pastries that covered her large, round oak table in the dining room as she rolled out the dough and prepared it for various fillings. There was never a recipe to use as a guide. She used a pinch of this, or a dash of that, and eventually produced a mouth watering baked good we considered to be fit for a king.

After she passed away, you would have thought that tradition would have been passed on to the only surviving daughter, but it didn't ever quite taste the same as memory recalled. Now, in 2009, as my mother rapidly becomes a member of the geriatric society, she no longer remembers how to boil water to make gelatin with canned fruit, let alone bake a pie from scratch. It's sad to watch the memory come and go, similar to the waxing and waning of the moon. Some days the memory is better than others.

Today's modern conveniences allow for a store bought crust to be filled with either canned fruit fillings, or fruit that happens to be in the peak of its growing season. Unless you are Julia Childs, or Rachel Ray, you probably follow the baking directions on the can of filling to produce a final product.

Whatever the outcome, it still makes the kitchen smell like someone has been busy enough to fill the air with pleasant aromas of homemade goods.

Eating the dessert is a personal experience. Do you eat the top crust, then the filling, before devouring the bottom crust? Do you eat the triangular shaped slice a bite of each layer at a time? Think about your preferences. Your mouth is probably watering now just thinking about downing a slice of home made pie.

One memory I will have of my folks enjoying eating pie during their late eighties and early nineties is the fact that they cut the entire pie into six pieces, because they couldn't eat eight!

BLUEBERRY BAGELS

As my parents age, I discover the physical attributes gradually change over the years. Eye sight is one vital sense that we rely on daily for accomplishing routine tasks. Since both parents have macular degeneration, upon researching the topic I learn that this particular medical problem is usually passed on to the daughter. Not a detail that I was overjoyed to learn.

With this problem, arrives the need for magnifying glasses for reading the newspaper, computer screen, phone book, television schedules, or menus when dining out. Not only are enlargers necessary for reading, but my mother should have one in hand for creating the grocery list, making phone calls, writing checks, or finding the left-over foods in the refrigerator.

This became more significant when she was preparing breakfast one Sunday morning. She announced we were having blueberry bagels, along with the preference of orange juice or coffee. Upon closer inspection by someone without macular degeneration, we soon discovered we were not having blueberry bagels, but bagels that had grown blue hair while being in the refrigerator longer than the recommended date on the packaging, and we were almost served moldy bagels that were no longer edible.

Frustrations caused by poor vision are more evident when dining in local restaurants. Lighting is never quite good enough, print on the menus is much too small, and the table is not one where they anticipated having seating. Again we have the complaint department. Since she seems to find a blunder with part of the meal, even if it wasn't the fault of the waitress or the chef, my mother manages to have a portion of the bill reduced, the entire meal removed from the bill, or receives a complementary dessert for problems voiced to the server. Dining out becomes a serious and sometimes embarrassing challenge!

I am convinced there is a photo of my mother hanging in every restaurant kitchen in the city, much like a wanted poster that hangs in a post office. The caption which identifies the photo would remind servers that it is their turn to wait on her. Someone else was the target of her wrath last time that restaurant was visited. Whatever the situation, that infamous magnifying glass was a critical piece of the puzzle. To the server's dismay at wherever the restaurant, it's a missing piece, but it probably wouldn't have made a difference.

House Cleaning Versus Clutter

Used aluminum foil perilously stacked in a frying pan on the left back burner of the stove, paper bags and plastic containers from delivered dinners by the nearby carry-out restaurant, stacks of empty containers from whipping cream, empty popcorn bags carefully lined with an empty bread wrapper stapled inside and awaiting "wet" garbage, or that last bite of chili stashed in a small container in the refrigerator are visible when you inspect the kitchen. It doesn't matter how many times the cleaning lady or I toss one or all of these items.

They magically reappear on the stove, kitchen sink, or in the fridge. Much like the blueberry bagels, items are kept "just in case" they may be of additional use, or for future consumption. The stove top was also a temporary resting place for a dead hydrangea prior to it making its way down the stairs to the basement shelf.

It's difficult to discern whether the need to keep used items instead of throwing them out after using them is a condition resulting from the depression of the 1920s, or if it's a lack of organizational skills. The rest of the house is similar in chaotic disorder. The attic and basement are strewn with boxes full of items that litter the floor. Some items are useful and just need to be stored away, so they are out of the foot path, and saved for future use. Other things are old, with crumbled, discolored pages and should be sent to the city land fill. Items have been deposited in one area or another of the residence, but could be donated to local charities so they could be of use to someone less fortunate.

The bedrooms and living room are not without their own untidiness. Unfinished pieces of sewing and knitting are boxed and stacked in both bedrooms. The pathway between the twin beds in their master bedroom is wide enough for walking, but dangerous for elderly unstable journeys to and from the bathroom during the night. Closed blinds make the room dark and uninviting. Stained clothing hangs in the closet, or is piled at the foot of both beds. On one night in particular, my mother complained about an uncomfortable night of sleep. She had slept on the edge of her single bed because there were too many clothes piled along the opposite side. Hanging up the clothes seemed to be a sensible idea, but also appeared to be out of the question.

The step-ladder from the garage stands alone in the corner behind the bedroom door. After use to repair the ceiling fan, it never made the trek back to the garage. The living room has boxes and baskets of mail received either recently, or during past years. Envelopes are arranged in various sized cardboard boxes by category or date. Most could be destroyed or placed in the trash. At any rate, it has become a navigational nightmare for elderly persons who must use a cane for stability.

Occasional visits by myself, or the regular bi-weekly visits by the hired cleaning agency result in frustration. The clutter apparent to visitors is unseen by the home owners. Two broken VCRs in the basement, the hidden microwave oven that sits on the hall closet floor, and two reclining chairs in the basement along with two more microwave ovens, are a few of the items that will not leave the premises. The question remains: "Why is it difficult for some people to let go of seemingly unusable items?"

Trash Police

Cleaning is a test of wills when visiting my parents, but there are times when insistence wins over resistance. Those blueberry bagels are not the only items in the fridge that need to go into the garbage. Again, the macular degeneration of both parents creates a challenge for items placed in the refrigerator as a bite sized portion of leftovers. Alzheimer's multiplies the problem as those bits of leftover meals are soon forgotten about and get pushed to the back of the refrigerator.

Their home town has what seems to me as ridiculous rules for putting out trash. Collections by the enormous trash eating vehicles are limited to once a week. Placement of bags containing garbage, collapsed boxes, paper products, or larger bulky items are staggered for pick ups scheduled by labeled "red" and "blue" weeks. Newspapers and boxes are to be wrapped, as one would meticulously tie up Christmas gifts, prior to be placed curbside for the Sunday midnight pick up. Some items are to be placed in black trash bags for designated "blue" weeks, while others are inserted into clear white garbage bags designated for recyclable items for alternate "red" pick up weeks. Due to the nature of the beast, I tend to grab the black bags and start tossing in garbage, wet or dry, as well as other clutter I can get away with throwing out without feeling like I've engaged in World War III.

As my parents were both raised in very strict homes during the depression, I find that they are guilt ridden when throwing away something that could possibly be useful next week, or even next month.

This is where the used pieces of aluminum foil, assorted plastic dishes from the corner carryout restaurant, or empty microwave popcorn bags meet their demise. According to the "trash rules" these items are not to be put together in the weekly trash. I have difficulty following these rules, and I know the "trash police" are not going to be rummaging through the bags to catch an unsuspecting individual who mixed the trash with items designated to go in the other color bag, or should be placed curbside the following week.

The basement, even though the dead plants have a home of their own in a far corner next to the washer and dryer, is amazing when you have to step over empty boxes that have been pitched down the stairway from the kitchen door access at the top of the stairs. Empty cereal boxes, useless styrofoam egg cartons, discarded cardboard containers that were used to ship those gift boxes of plants or cookies, or a variety of packages that once contained bags of mix for cake mixes or au graten potatoes litter the floor at the foot of the stairs. These containers could go into the weekly trash bags, but they are given a good heave to land wherever at the bottom of the stairs, in hopes that eventually they make their way to an empty red or blue trash bag that gets set out at curbside for the appropriate Sunday evening truck to haul away.

During the normal course of events my folks put out one or two trash bags per week. When I am there, I can manage to sneak out an average of fifteen bags per visit. The longer the visit, the more bags I can dispose of each week. My all time record during one particular visit was seventeen bags of discarded trash. Here again, to avoid interaction that would appear to be synonymous with World War III, I am forced to enlist the assistance of neighbors who didn't mind a few bags being added to their curb side area for pick up. It looked like they were on a cleaning binge, and fortunately for me they had no problem at all with more bags than usual being in stacked front of their home. Trash police or not, it all is divided for distribution to the same city dump on "blue" weeks, or to the recycling center on "red" weeks, depending on the color of the bag scheduled to be placed at the edge of the curb!

HARD COOKIES

Each manufacturing company in the United States has a complaint department where consumers can report irregularities in products received that did not measure up to the recipients expectations. Buying gifts for my mother and father takes on a whole new meaning since it is difficult, at best, to find something with which she, in particular, does not find fault. Distance also increases the optional use of making purchases on the internet so shipping more readily accomplished by the click of the computer mouse.

Over the past few years, it has become a painstaking task to find new items that satisfy the expectations of a gift for birthdays, Mother's Day, Father's Day, wedding anniversaries, or Christmas. Gifts are usually met with repugnance.

One would think gifts were damaged, the incorrect size, or arrived with some other malady, but the one that met with the most outrageous reproach was the package of cookies ordered for one particular Christmas delivery. Since the old folks love sweets, and regularly ask the neighbor who takes them for the weekly Saturday outing to stop so they can purchase day-old cookies from the corner convenience store, you'd expect that a delivery of a festively wrapped tub of 12 dozen special order cookies would suffice.

I was amazed to learn that when the cookies arrived at the front door via the UPS truck, after opening the parcel and consuming a few, a phone call to complain was placed to the company. Why?

She felt compelled to alert the customer service representative that the cookies were too hard to chew. Besides that fact, she asked the cookie company representative what were they supposed to do with 12 dozen cookies!

Patience must be the word of the day for customer service representative who meet the fury of an angry, old woman who had just received a container of hard cookies! Thankfully, the representative from the un-named cookie company explained the cookies could be warmed in a micro-wave oven for a few seconds, and magically they would become somewhat softer for chewing. That seemed to do the trick, but it makes me wonder if some companies have their customer representative keep a log of reasons for complaints, so they too can write a book about such nonsense.

One needs to remember two rules of ordering online: (1) Once you find a company that completely satisfies the recipients expectations, put them in your files for future reference. (2) You cannot control old people and their need to complain about something. Grumbling seems to be an elderly person phenomenon.

I am also learning that there is a trend that involves elderly people who are now displaying signs of elder rage. This is more apparent in my mother, who can change attitudes and behaviors more quickly than you can flip a coin. Knowledge of elder rage does not make it easier to deal with, but when one understands this phenomenon it increases variety of ways the adult child can react to situation. The most common response would be to fight fire with fire. That counter response of madness only prolongs the rage of the elderly person. What seems to be a personal attack on the adult child needs to be met with an attitude of coolness and patience. Speaking from experience, that's not the easiest thing to do. Critical attacks create a situation for the adult child that are the basis of frustration and create thoughts of reprisal. Those thoughts prolong a prickly state of affairs.

I have learned to expect the unexpected. Elder rage is responsible for creating situations beyond the adult child's control. Walking away from the situation is not an option, but stepping back and observing the circumstances of the moment as an outsider give a sense of detachment required for everyone concerned.

It is difficult to comprehend that an innocent cookie is reason for alarm, but with the elderly recipient also having moments that lack lucidity, even a hard cookies will cause feedback with seemingly unexplainable, malicious retorts.

To Drive, Or Not To Drive

Macular degeneration not only causes concerns in the area of reading, but it also creates dangerous situations for drivers. My dad was first to relinquish his driver's license, but it took the assistance of their family doctor to convince my mother to forego the ability of driving their personal auto. Doing research about older people and the driving ages I learned there is a minimum driving age, but most states do not have a maximum driving age where someone is legally required to stop driving.

It is amazing to see their car today riddled with dents and scratches. Even though my father gave up his license without a fight, he felt compelled to back the car out of the garage, or pull it in after the neighbor drove it and them to the grocery store and back for their weekly shopping spree. The worst scenario was the day Dad stepped on the gas instead of the brake, and managed to drive the car through the back of the garage knocking the back wall about two feet off the footer. The crashing noise brought several neighbors scurrying out of their homes, like rats with their tails on fire, to check the destruction to back wall of the garage, the car, as well as the possibility of injury to my dad.

Fortunately, the damage to the car and garage were worse than injury to the driver. It took one of the neighbors to back the car out of the damaged structure. A tow truck had to be called to use a large chain attached to the back of his truck to draw the back of the garage in and realign it on the foundation. Another handy man was hired to replace the broken window so the summer rains would not damage other contents stored in the garage. The dented front hood of the car now matches the back hatch of the mini van since he also managed to run into the side of the garage door when backing the car out of the garage on another occasion.

My mother, on the other hand, only had one minor accident involving another car. That minor fender bender was enough to convince the doctor to discuss the end of her driving career with her during a routine office visit. He was instrumental in convincing her she should give up that level of independence. That's probably the most difficult decision we see older parents have to make. It's one of the last points of independence they have in their mature years.

Taxi cabs, neighbors, and the local mini-bus named the "Lift" are all modes of reliable transportation at this point in time. At least the roads are safer for them and others. Interesting to observe older drivers who are in their late 80s and early 90s still behind the wheels on our nation's highways. It makes one question how quick elderly drivers' reflexes are, and how good their eye sight might be. Will we be as reluctant to relinquish our independence?

PHONE SOLICITATIONS

Elderly people are usually more gullible when it comes to sales people calling in an attempt to solicit donations for a charity, locally or nationally based. Depending on who answers my parent's phone, they might be on the receiving end of spewed wrath, or if the mood is one of chattiness they could hear my mother's life story.

I know this because my second husband considered himself a jokester. Upon learning my folks had been to a local fast food restaurant and were dissatisfied with their meal, he called, disguised his voice, and pretended to be a vice-president of the company in question. This is where the gullibility came into play. His promise as a company representative to send coupons for free replacement meals to the restaurant was believed hook, line, and sinker. Not only did she respond positively with gratitude for the invented follow up call, but she proceeded to inform him of my first husband's escapades, the fact that she and my father liked husband number two better than husband number one, where I lived, what I did for an occupation, where my two marries sons lived, and exactly how old she and my dad were at that point in time.

After witnessing this event, not once, but twice, I conveyed my concerns to her regarding her friendly banter with whomever was on the other end of the phone line. Her unrelenting trust in people who call their home number is very unsettling to me. I listened to another one of these calls when I visited with them for a few days. In questioning my mother as to who she was talking to, why she was providing personal details, and how she knew who was calling, her reply was the lady who called "sounded nice" and knew her first name, so she felt comfortable talking with the caller. Fortunately, the caller wasn't asking for banking information.

It is next to impossible to convince my mother that in the twenty-first century people have access to a computer and have the capability to find information at their fingertips. Phone numbers, addresses, names, ages, and employment status are yours for the click of the computer mouse. The trust conveyed to total strangers who "seem" nice on the phone, could be a legitimate sales person, or a burglar who is calling from a cell phone and is sitting in a car parked just down the street.

My only hope is their phone number registered with the "Do Not Call" list will help eliminate some of those unsolicited phone calls.

DEAD PLANTS

Dead plants seem to be closely related to the hard cookie problem. Even ordering live plants from the internet based catalogue to be delivered for special occasions has its drawbacks. Once again, best intentions can go awry when the older adult is receiving a gift you anticipated would be graciously received.

As my brother used to say, "That's what you get for having expectations!"

Ordering a live plant for a birthday gift was a bit of a problem, after the fact. The proverbial phone call to the company customer service rep was made to get directions on watering procedures for this plant. The plant and its striking blue blossoms was gorgeous when it arrived. It didn't last long since the directions heard during the phone conversation on proper care and watering, were not the same directions that appeared on a the piece of scrap paper that lay on the kitchen table amongst the clutter.

Watering the plant once a week was translated into watering the plant once a day. This not only caused the plant to die within ten days, but it also resulted in a second phone call to the unfortunate customer service person who was on the receiving end of the irate conversation. Luckily, the company was gracious enough to replace the plant, even though it was not damaged in shipment, nor was it their fault that the perfectly beautiful hydrangea had succumbed to overwatering.

You also have to ask yourself about the second plant. Did it fall into the same demise as the first hydrangea? Of course it did! Now we have two dead plants. Do they get tossed in the trash, as most normal people would expect? (Here we are again with the expectations!) No! They get taken down to the basement, forever to be set on shelves that have now become dead plant heaven. These two plants join numerous other dead plants, dried up flowers from anniversaries, shriveled up funeral arrangements that were taken home for sentimental reasons, or the lone dead, shriveled up Christmas poinsettia that holds the place of honor on the top shelf.

OLD WHEAT PENNIES

It is interesting to look back on the history of the Unites States, and discover why Abraham Lincoln is on the front of the copper penny, and how often the back of the same coin has undergone design changes throughout the years. Finding a penny on the ground as you go about your travels usually makes you think of someone, or possibly triggers another recollection about your childhood, or the childhood rhyme about seeing a penny, picking it up and all day long having good luck.

My most vivid memory of not one, but thousands of pennies involves someone being shot in the head, as was Lincoln, but this person did not make as large a claim to his fame as Lincoln did years ago. Little did our family realize that my brother had collected pennies for years and stored them in empty check book boxes in the bedroom located in the basement of his three story home. The majority of these pennies were "old wheat" pennies with Lincoln's profile on the front of each penny, along with the two shafts of wheat stamped on the back of each one cent piece of copper.

After a mock shooting on a televised show involving a felony, you see police place yellow crime tape around the perimeter of an area to keep out unwanted people who might contaminate the scene. It is interesting to note that television depicts the police as they seemingly ransack a home looking for clues that would give an indication a person was indeed a criminal with intent to harm others. The individuals who are responsible for searching the premises appear to have no conscience or regard to the private possessions of the person they are investigating. They dump out dresser drawers of contents on to the floor, turn over pillows on furniture, rifle through closets, and leave no stone unturned in order to find evidence to use for a possible conviction.

It was after this invasion by the police department that we discovered although there were numerous boxes of these collector's items, they disregarded valuable things in their search for evidence. Not only was the family in shock over what has happened to their family member, but they are left with the disarray of the chaos the police left in the house. When the bedlam subsided, the coins were counted, carefully checked for dates and mint marks, and placed in collector's cards for those left behind. Countless hours of sorting and categorizing all of the old wheat pennies did not help lessen the agonizing loss.

LOSS OF A BROTHER AND FRIEND

Eighteen months ago, seems like only yesterday,

A friend phoned, she was sorry to say......,

"Shots had been fired in the neighborhood,

Two neighbors were critical; it didn't look good."

A year long fight was coming to an end,

The senseless feud, over childish things again and again.

Several days of anguish for the families of the two,

Spent in a hospital over looking a metro zoo.

One family traveled by plane from afar,

The other one's family only traveled by car.

Doctors and nurses spend countless hours,

In a room where no one could even send flowers.

The families each kept a vigil all through the night.

The outcome would have neither of the men end up all right.

Who would have expected either one to be shot,

"Why did they fight?" was the question each family thought.

One man would live, the other would die,

Neither family understood, as hard as they'd try.

One family struggles to make ends meet.

The other relinquished their son to self -defeat.

Peace and contentment followed for the one who is missed.

There is no real living. The survivor can't make a fist!

Fighting is such a ridiculous, childish plight.

One took his own life in the middle of the night.

Senseless Acts of Violence

If you or a loved one is involved in education, whether it be as a student or staff member of a school, we all worry about the increase in the number of school shootings, as well as random acts of violence in our neighborhoods.

There are numerous unnecessary displays of anger and frustration that impact pre-schools and extend to university campuses. We worry about being shot, or a family member being killed by senseless firings of ammunition, but how many of us are concerned about the fact that one of our family members would be the shooter?

Four years ago on a relatively quiet, summer evening, I never would have imagined that my brother would have been involved in an act of violence. When I answered the phone, I expected to hear his girlfriend's voice and to become engaged in a normal, friendly conversation. Shock, disbelief, and horror are the only words that come to mind as I relive that life altering event. My brother had gone to his neighbor's home, shot and wounded the father of the family, returned to his driveway and ended his own life. Days and weeks of turmoil ensued.

The focus of these tragedies is on the loss of the innocent victims, as it should be; however, the loss is just as great for the family of the culprit who committed the horrific deed. In the days following the crime, the culprit's family asks the same question that everyone asks. Why?

The culprit's family not only deals with their personal loss, but they also deal with the fact that other lives have been ended without regard for age, race, or creed. Understanding the process is difficult, at best. It is unnecessary to end the lives of others.

We live in a society the embraces freedom of speech, religion, and ability to buy weapons. We also have a generation of people who are on medications that alter mental states. Those medications mask the underlying depression haunting many Americans. Not everyone who is taking medication for depression is at risk for committing a dastardly crime, but when a person is taking a prescribed dosage, then suddenly stops, or enhances the medication with alcohol the combinations become lethal.

Do you look for warning signs? Probably not! Even if you do, they are difficult to identify. My brother would have been the first to tell a someone who was struggling with drug or alcohol dependency and abuse to seek help, straighten out their life style, and become a responsible citizen. Never in my wildest dreams did I ever anticipate my brother deliberately trying to kill another human being. His own life was not threatened. He was not defending himself, nor his property. Such an act was, and still is, unbelievable.

No one can ever predict the reactions to such crimes in our society, or how you will respond when they will impact you personally. There are no answers to questions about the senseless taking of someone else's life. The loss of a child is a parent's worst nightmare. When the shooter is your family member, the loss is compounded by the knowledge that your child or sibling committed such a heinous crime. We will never have an understanding regarding why someone caused these unfortunate fatalities.

The best thing we can do is show compassion to the victim's families, both the innocent and the guilty! Each of these individuals is someone's child.

This was an article printed in my local newspaper in response to the editor's question of why there is an increase in shootings in our neighborhoods and on school campuses. People who listen to the news broadcast, or read about shootings in the local newspapers usually only consider the families who were killed by the gun man. Seldom do folks think about the family of the shooter and their loss.

GENTLE GIANTS

Unconditional love, security, companionship. Those are usually three qualities that you would expect to receive from your mother, but there are times in your life when you will find these qualities somewhere else. Woof, woof, woof, would be the sounds you hear when you knock on my front door. This thundering bark comes from not one dog, but from two gentle giants. Great Danes and St. Bernards are not your usual small breed of dog that you can pick up. These dogs are enormous in size. You don't even have to bend over to pet them. Let me explain to you why these dogs offer so much love, a feeling of safety, and friendship.

Providing love for anyone without expecting something in return, or loving them no matter how they treat you is unconditional love. Usually, that's the love a child receives from a parent. Animals are similar in nature. They love you, even if you treat them badly. That happy tail wagging the moment you step foot in the house is a good indication that your pet is glad to see you. You can be gone for five minutes, or five hours, and the response is still the same. Did you ever have what seemed to be a yard of tongue run across your face? With a Great Dane or a St. Bernard, sometimes it seems like their tongues are endless, especially after they just got a drink of water. Yuk, sometimes it's from the bathroom commode!!!

In this day and age, home security systems are in one of every seven homes in the neighborhood. In my home, the security system weighs about 260 pounds all together, and they have thundering barks that sound loud enough to wake the dead, and two sets of teeth. I doubt any burglar would want to meet up with them in a dark room. Dogs have much better hearing than humans, so once they become accustomed to the normal, everyday noises in and around the house, they hear anything unusual. Their barks even send the pizza delivery person to the edge of the driveway. All of a sudden, he isn't sure if he is delivering dinner, or if he could end up being eaten alive. I love living in a house where I feel safe.

Alone? I'm never alone when I am at home. Every time I move, I have two cold, wet noses that follow my every move. You'd think they'd figure out that I'm only going into the next room, but just incase I get lost, or can't find what I'm looking for, each of these goofy dogs has to follow me where ever I go. It's nice to have the companionship, but when the phone rings, I am the last one to get to it. It's not as if they were going to answer it, but they know I'm going to move when they hear that ding-a-ling of the telephone. My Great Dane loves to watch television with me in the evening. She has even calculated where she has to park her butt on the couch, so she can roll back, and land with her head strategically placed in my lap. Not only are they good company for me, but they also provide companionship to each other during the day when I am at school. Companionship is important to animals and humans.

Love from family, friends, or pets is important. In this day and age, it's great to feel safe and secure. You can find someone to talk to most places you go, but it's comforting to have someone to talk to at home. I can tell my dogs any thing, and they won't go out and tell the neighbor's dog. My secrets are safe with them. There are other things that are important in life, but you will never find anyone as trustworthy and loyal as your dog, man's best friend. As I have explained love, security, and companionship to you, my best friend is barking in my ear! Must be time for her to eat?

In order to describe my childhood pets to a classroom full of sixth graders, this was a modeled five paragraph expository essay. Growing older has become an adventure. There were many dogs, cats, and rabbits that came and went in our lives as children. People who have animals that provide love, companionship, and security are alleged to live longer than those who do not care for pets. As I watch my parents become octogenarians, then nonagenarians, I wonder what my sons will deal with as I become elderly. My middle son jests that he and I are not far away from that situation!

GROWING UP – A VISIT BACK TO CHILDHOOD

Growing up, graduating from high school, and getting married are all examples of major changes in a person's life. Throughout your life time, things happen that may or may not be out of your control, but they shape your personality and destiny along the path of living. Events that cause you to think about your survival of your personal being are the most memorable. Your next important area of learning and growing involves the emotions. Finally, information required for general knowledge is least important of the three learning essentials.

Babies emerge into children, who turn into adolescents, and eventually reach the age of independence. Throughout the first eighteen years of life, children learn by trial and error. Usually, they don't like to listen to advice from grown-ups; they want and need to make their own mistakes that hopefully will become lessons for growth. One of life's lessons I learned when I was six years old was that you never add water to the gas tank of a car. Seems like a no-brainer, but my younger brother and I were only trying to help, or so we thought.

Our father, along with the assistance of our maternal grandfather, began the process of constructing a cement block building which would become a temporary home while the next phase of building the house that would become our actual residence located the same acre of property was taking place.

One particular summer afternoon my younger brother and I were bored!

A wheelbarrow that our father had used to mix cement to slather between the concrete blocks stood in the driveway unattended. Since we were in the country, an old fashioned pump was the only source of water. Boredom is the mother of invention. Water was pumped from the well, poured into the wheelbarrow, and then mixed together until it appeared to be the proper consistency. Looking at our mixture, the car became the perfect place to put the concoction to good use.

I recall the events that followed more clearly than how we got the gas cap off, and poured the water filled with particles of cement into the gas tank, but it was a memorable evening. Our mother had been at work all day as a sales clerk in a local department store. Hours passed during the afternoon, so we took Grandpa home for dinner with Grandma, and we continued our journey to pick up Mom. Hmmmmm, the car stalled about three miles from our destination. Dad had no idea about what was wrong with the car. He and a passing good citizen pushed the sluggish auto to the curb side, and we waited on the corner for the next bus to arrive. Mom was really surprised to see us wave to her from our seats near the window, as she stood on the corner. She had expected to be picked up in the car. After boarding the bus and sitting down on the empty seat next to our father, she questioned him extensively about the car. Where was it? What happened?

Did he have any idea what was wrong with it? Did Grandpa get home okay? What were we going to do for dinner? Question after question remained a mystery without concrete answers.

The next day, Dad was able to make arrangements to get the car towed to a repair shop so they could inspect the car for possible problems with explainable solutions. Wow, were my brother and I in trouble! Our gas station activity caused the cement particles to clog the gas line. No gas, the car won't run, period. I have no idea how much it cost for the replacement and repairs of the entire gas line of the car, but that learning experience taught me never to add water to a gas tank of a car again. I don't recall the punishment, but I'm sure it wasn't fun!

Graduation from high school, attendance at a small Ohio college, and getting my first teaching position were what I considered uneventful, especially after the gas station game my brother and I had created. Attending classes, reading textbooks, taking exams, and traveling home periodically to have a decent home cooked meal seemed like normal procedures for any college student. I have a personal belief that people come and go in your life as they are needed. That was certainly true in college. I never kept in contact with anyone who attended college with me. My first teaching position didn't create any life long friends, but I did meet the son of a teacher in my building who had returned from service in the Army, and he eventually became my first husband. People come and go in your life, and that relationship continued for fifteen years. Even today, although that marriage produced three children, there is no contact with that side of the family by my sons or me.

Optimistically, when someone marries, they are mature enough to handle situations that arise. Most couples argue over the handling of money, how to discipline their children, or something that is important to one spouse, but not the other. As people, single or married, grow and change over the years, ideas or convictions from their youth become more deeply embedded, or change with various situations presented. When, and if, the marriage "runs out of gas", so to speak, it ends in divorce. To this day, my parents have been married for sixty-five years. Even now, they recall the "gas station" escapade involving the cement.

Change is inevitable, sometimes difficult to anticipate and predict, but change is a valuable part of life. There will be individuals who will enter your life, and then be gone when their use has ended. Some will move away to another city, or they may change jobs or careers, or some will pass over to the next world so they can watch over us as guardian angels. Life is full of changes, some slight and hardly noticeable, while others are traumatic and alter your life forever. The most difficult change in life to accept is one of letting go! No one ever prepares you for that change while you are growing up! Letting go forces one to encounter lessons of survival, strong emotions, and more general knowledge than you ever anticipate.

This is another example of an expository essay for my sixth grade class. As a veteran teacher who has forty years of classroom experience, I strongly believe it is important to let them know that good writing involves personal experiences. Not everyone has a "happily-ever-after" life as you see in the movies. Life is not a Disney film where the good guy always wins. In their declining years, my parents seldom reminisce about life when my brother and I were growing up. The gas station recollection is one of the few stories they remind me of now as an adult child.

CHANGES

A cup of coffee, the morning news, a phone call from a friend! Usually these components would be the beginning of a somewhat normal day in the life of a mother. Still clad in pajamas, I sipped on my first cup of coffee. The drone of the announcer's voice on television was heard in the back ground. The phone rang. It was the car dealership sales person who was inquiring as to what kind of new car I was considering for my upcoming purchase. The discussion ensued: leather or upholstered seats, four doors versus two doors, six cylinder engine versus four; and most important, the choices of interior and exterior colors.

The coffee still simmered as the conversation regarding the details continued. The first cup of coffee was consumed, and a second cup of coffee was poured, doctored with cream and sugar to enhance the flavor of the bitter bean taste. News continued to be projected from the broadcaster's voice as he told of traffic, weather, and sports events. The phone conversation about the car was still foremost in my mind. Multi-tasking is a mother's strong suit, so drinking coffee, listening to the news, and the phone conversation all continued for a few minutes.

I listened to the news on television and heard about an auto accident that had closed both east and west bound lanes of traffic on Pine Ridge Road at 7:30 that morning.

The thought immediately ran through my mind that my youngest son had left earlier than that, so he should have cleared the area prior to the accident and was well on his way to the high school for summer classes. A knock on the door interrupted the coffee, news, as well as the phone call. Looking out the front window, I noticed a car in the driveway. This was not a regular car of someone who may be lost and was looking for a specific address. It was one from the Florida Highway Patrol. Abruptly ending my phone call, still clad in black silky pajamas, I went to answer the door. As I walked across the living room to the front door, a million thoughts raced through my mind. Were they looking for an escaped criminal who was possibly seen in the neighborhood, had my husband been in an accident, had something happened that involved my oldest son? I knew my middle son was still asleep in the bedroom, so he was fine. How many thoughts can a person have in a few seconds?

As the door was opened, one of the officers asked if I had a son named Jason. After an affirmative response from me, he told me there had been an accident. Of course, my reply was to ask where he was and suggest that I would go get him. Never in a mother's wildest dreams would I expect to hear the words, "I'm sorry, he didn't make it!" The echo of those words sends shivers down a mother's spine. Seconds seemed like hours.

The officers entered the living room and asked if there was anyone else home. Think! I had to think! Yes, my middle son was still in bed. I don't remember what I said to him as I opened the bedroom door to wake him with the news of the accident, but he can tell me what I uttered. I was in shock!! Neither of us could comprehend the situation. I recalled the news I had heard earlier spoken by the broadcaster! There was an accident on Pine Ridge Road. My immediate thought was he had made it past the accident. He hadn't made it past the accident! He and his car were the accident!!

That first morning phone call about the new car was replaced by phone calls to family and friends. Friends were so important at this time of grief and overwhelming loss. The Florida Highway Patrol officers stayed and made several calls to have my husband return home from work, and to find someone to stay with us. One friend arrived and throughout the next few hours made 75 phone calls in an attempt to locate family, who all lived in various parts of the country.

My life as a mother had abruptly changed forever. Did I want a cup of coffee? No, I couldn't even think of eating anything. That day I listened to the afternoon news as they announced the loss of a seventeen year old Naples High School senior. Phone calls were coming regularly as family and friends heard the news, made plans, and called to see how we were coping. All of those calls were screened by several friends who spent the next few days at the house. Life has many changes. Some of them are within our control, but some of them are out of our control. Those changes that are out of our control are the hardest to understand, and learn to deal with on a daily basis!

We don't understand the lessons we are presented in life until we see how we can assist someone with the same circumstances. I was able to tell my parents about what experiences life might possibly hand them as they also dealt with the loss of their youngest child. Although my brother was 55 years old when he passed on to the next life, it was still the loss of a child. Parents aren't supposed to outlive their children.

They would soon encounter holidays, birthdays, and anniversaries that now would be celebrated without their son. The hardest day to deal with is Mother's Day, or Father's Day. It's interesting how your mind decides how your body will react. The anticipation of the day is just as difficult to deal with as the actual day itself. I watch as my parents deal with the day, similarly to my own dealings of a multitude of emotions. Each celebrated day seems to bring with it times of depression, physical sickness, loss of appetite, or memories of happier times. All of these emotions bring a string of overwhelming feelings that are difficult for the outsider to understand. The loss of a child is something you never get over. You just learn to live with the horrific loss.

Little did I realize this loss of my youngest son would be paralleled six years later by the death of my younger brother. Lessons learned that surrounded one loss would be recalled to assist my parents in the same sorrowful experience.

MEDICATIONS

Alzheimer's disease coupled with macular degeneration creates a challenge for elderly patients and their loved ones. After spending six weeks with my parents as my house guests, it was apparent that a new system needed to be devised to assist with the daily chore of preparing medications. This morning ritual became increasingly more frustrating, more than ever for my mother who was the recipient of new medications after a hospital stay in my home town, followed by a second week long admission to her hospital upon their return home the next week.

Not being able to read labels on the medicine bottles, along with not remembering which medication was to be taken at what time of day, made it necessary for a system of labels. Each bottle of tablets was assigned a number which coincided with a number on a sheet that named the medication, dosage, and times to be taken during the day. Use of a computer to document this made it easy to create a page with large, readable print that could be understood even without the use of a magnifying glass. A permanent black marker was used to identify the pill container caps so numbers were more readable as well.

Organization became the key to helping with proper medications being administered on a daily basis without outside assistance. I find this another link to the independence they are so eager to maintain.

With each parent, the computer generated lists allow them to have medications at their fingertips, and also provides an immediate list of medications and dosages for emergency medical personnel who may be summoned in the event of an accident or sudden illness.

The one lasting concern is how to deal with panic which sets in when there is an emergency. Alzheimer's causes serious forgetfulness in someone who used to react during an emergency with reasonable expectations, but now cannot recall who should be contacted in the event of a stroke or heart attack experienced by a spouse. In my case, I am fortunate that neighbors are usually called, and they can step in to help with situations that provide cause for alarm.

DEALING WITH DOCTORS AND HOSPITALS

Allow me to digress in this chapter. Learning to deal with doctors and hospital began when my youngest son was killed in an automobile accident. In reading the autopsy report and talking with one of the paramedics who worked on him at the scene of the auto accident one July morning, I began to learn the medical jargon necessary to discuss all that was happening in what seemed like a life time.

During the course of the next several years, I would also find myself dealing with my current husband's numerous hospital stays, and another son's motorcycle accident which resulted in him being air lifted by a medical flight helicopter from the scene to one of the local hospitals. I soon learned that in dealing with the tragic loss of the youngest son, my mind refused to cooperate when discussing time lines for a variety of medicines, probable outcomes for many surgeries, details suggested by heart specialists or infection specialists, rotation of nurses, along with expectations for long term physical therapy, and what seemed like was an endless routine of changing dressings on wounds. With so many details to keep track of, I enlisted the help of a stenographer's note book, and kept pages upon pages of notes that could be revisited at a moments notice to recall and review doctor's comments, names of medicines, and descriptions of daily care by the nursing staff when I made the treks to the hospital rooms of whomever happened to be admitted for hospital care at the time.

One unwavering belief is that every thing happens for a reason. After countless hospital visits to my son, as well as my husband at that time in history, my knowledge increased with every visit, and the stenographer's note book graduated to a multi-chapter notebook divided into a personal section for each of several members of the immediate family. Another interesting fact observed in hospitals was if a visitor appears as if they know where they are going in a medical facility, then they are seldom questioned about where it is they wish to go.

The medical knowledge I had gained over the course of seven years was even more valuable when my younger brother became a suicide victim. Now the leather folder required insertion of a new triple sectioned notebook that would record more data from yet another hospital in different state. The details recorded during previous hospital visits, read, and re-read over the previous years provided an authoritative impression that made my brother's brain surgeon inquire about my medical background. The fact that I was able to ask intelligent questions regarding pending surgery to remove bone and bullet fragments from the shattered frontal lobe, caused the surgical staff seriously considered that I was a member of a nursing staff in another city.

The difficulty with this hospital visit was it would result in making life and death decisions. Faced with letting go of their youngest child and only son, what seemed like a long time actually was a span of fewer than twenty-four hours. Once again, faced with a grave situation that would result in making funeral arrangements, notification of family and friends, it was my undaunting task to make sure everything was organized and final details were resolved quickly and thoroughly. As difficult as it was, the situation was easier to contend with than making arrangement for my own son.

These details surrounding the death of my brother were influential in successfully convincing my parents to contact their family attorney so living wills and Power of Attorney forms could be signed, as well as each of them drawing up their Last Will and Testaments.

Taking notes during hospital stays for loved ones has become somewhat of a ritual. During the past three years that spiral bound notebook inserted in the leather folder has been used to document conversations about several surgeries, and also a multitude of visits to a handful of doctors for heart problems, colon and skin cancer check-ups, eye operations, and a variety of concerns stemming from changes in heart rhythms to a collection of a gross amount of wax in an ear canal. The well-known files provide an anthology of needed medical information in a variety of situations.

THE PROVERBIAL CHRISTMAS LETTER

We've all received letters in Christmas cards from people who enjoy sharing what's gone on during the past 12 months. Throughout the years, mailing of lengthy Christmas letters became the norm. It couldn't just be a Christmas card with a snappy holiday greeting. It had to be a calendar listing of the most miniscule details for all to read, or ignore, whatever the case happened to be. Not all recipients wanted to read the details for daily life from my folk's calendar for the year. This idea was difficult to convey to my folks who expected everyone to want to know what they did on a daily basis throughout the year. Eventually, it was necessary to take the bull by the horns, and complete the typing, revising, and printing of the yearly task. The letters took on a professional design with use of computer programs.

Taking over the task of creating the letter meant the daily items describing going to church, the doctor's office, grocery shopping, daily menus, and the like, flowed into recounting monthly events for the first several years. The longest seasonal greeting was the summary of sixty years of marriage. It contained sixty photos each with an adjective phrase to depict and note many of the celebrated years. From that year forward the monthly itinerary gave way to a shortened poetic version with a few family pictures. The most recent holiday greeting contained a shorter poem, and went from a few photos to two significant photos.

It's been over ten years since I began the yearly ritual of creating the annual holiday greeting. For all practical purposes this year, the proverbial Christmas message will take on a new look, with one photo, and a couple of quick lines conveying a personal touch letting family and friends know they are both still alive and well.

Computers make life easier to store photos, accumulate rough drafts, edit and revise details, print cards and address lists. This makes life easier for me as I continue to create such master pieces. At 93 years of age, my father has embraced this age of technology by playing solitaire, or even sending an occasional e-mail to family and friends; however, my mother is afraid of the mouse!

I still have the honor of completing the annual Christmas letter, but this year it will be shorter and sweeter! My motto will be: "A picture is worth a thousand words!"

DEMENTIA VERSUS ALZHEIMER'S

Illnesses are not always something that is visible to the observer, whether it be a family member, friend, or member of the medical community. This affliction usually attacks the elderly in varying stages.

I have been present for doctor's visits with both parents, but the ones that are most incomprehensible are my mother's routine evaluation appointments. For short periods of time averaging approximately ten to fifteen minutes, the patient exhibiting signs of any stage of dementia can be personable, coherent, and friendly. It's during longer discussions that the true personality appears and the elder rage becomes more apparent to an observer. Doctors and nurses can be greeted with pleasantries and seemingly appropriate answers to queries about health and well being. Longer visits require a back up assistant to make sure there is a clear and concise message that is adequately communicated about concerns for the patient that indicate reality rather than fiction.

The resemblance of normalcy for brief periods of time gives the doctor an impression that all is well, when quite the opposite is true. Once again, the proverbial notebook with pages laden in ink that record details depicting more accurate events of daily routines provides a better picture of the patient's behaviors.

Dementia creates a misrepresentation of the facts to medical care givers, especially in the event of an emergency situation. One situation where my father required the ambulance was met with my mother not providing his medical information, but instead she gave them her listing of medicines and a verbal dialogue describing her afflictions. This was not one of her more lucid moments, and the situation could have had negative results if one of the neighbors had not been present to take charge of the situation and redirect their questions to collect information regarding the proper patient.

Dementia also creates an atmosphere compared to one of dealing with a child instead of an adult. The behaviors revert to those similar to a little kid who worries about someone hiding under the bed at night, or even added exuberance of an upcoming birthday.

Dealing with medical staffs, or just day to day living, the status of the elderly person's mind is critical to their care. At this point in time, my mother's biggest concern is what will happen to her once her spouse is gone. She worries, as does a child, about tomorrow, or the day after, or next week. She has forgotten that funeral arrangements are finalized. There is not much one can say or do to alleviate the worries. There is little reassurance in her mind that she will be provided for in the event of his passing first.

Neighbors

The distance between Florida and Pennsylvania causes problems now that my folks are declining in their activities which created independence for so many years. As the only daughter who still spends ten months out of the year fulfilling requirements of her teaching career, time that passes between visits is usually longer than anticipated.

In my parent's endeavors to maintain their independence in their own home, it becomes difficult to know how much to insist on moving them to an assisted living facility, moving to Florida to live in my home, or to have in home health assistance. Since none of those options provide any agreeable solution, they are content to remain in their own residence. Seems we have not arrived at the stage where there is going to be a definite answer readily available.

Fortunately for all concerned, there are two special neighbors who have become regular overseers for serious events, or help by coming to their aid for weekly necessities. Being members of the baby-boomer era and having elderly parents themselves, or recently having lost older parents, they are very understanding of the situation. Phone calls between Florida and Pennsylvania keep lines of communication open so those of us in the baby boomer era can all be kept apprized of what's happening with the geriatric generation.

For the past five years, under the circumstances, it has been wonderful to have devoted neighbors who have helped them through many situations. Grocery shopping outings every Saturday morning, accompanying the folks to pay city taxes, trips to the doctor's offices, travels to their other property to check on yet another situation brewing there, or just checking on them daily to see how they are doing in general makes my life much easier from 1500 miles away. I can never repay their generosity and concern for people to whom they aren't even related.

As the Alzheimer's and/or Dementia continue to deteriorate the mind, there are days when my mother doesn't recognize her neighbors. It will be interesting to see how the near future takes twists and turns that may or may not be unexpected.

Funeral Arrangements

Goals are important for many people. Within the past two years, my goal was to discuss funeral arrangements for each parent, make sure those arrangements were in writing with a local funeral home, and have their arrangement pre-paid so at the appropriate time, their wishes would be fulfilled.

This was a delicate situation, at best, but with the help of several people in their community who offered advice, it was a completed goal by the end of the year. It took several months of discussions to get my parents to agree to having funeral arrangements in writing. Once they agreed, it was a challenge to get the funeral director they wanted to write their plans for each of them. After getting the folks to agree, I was able to contact a funeral director to make a home visit. Neither parent drives their car, so fortunately, it was convenient for someone to go to them.

The first problem encountered was that my father did not agree with the choice of funeral homes, although that particular original one scheduled was my understanding. Cancelling that appointment, discussing a different funeral home, making another appointment for a home visit was an undertaking, but do-able. When my brother passed away, one of the local funeral directors sent a note of condolence since she was acquainted with him and had attended the same Indiana based college as he during his undergraduate years.

Fortunately, that gave my folks a personal connection and with her guidance the funeral arrangements for each parent were finalized.

The second problem was arranging for payments. Alzheimer's disease impacts the memory, so it became a series of constant reminders that payments needed to be made according to the schedule they had agreed upon with the director. Over the course of six months, the capability of paying via check drafts from their checking account over the internet, all funds were delivered to the appropriate sources. At the time of their passing, life will be easier for the one left behind, as well as for me. All arrangements have been made according to their wishes, so making those difficult decisions has already been completed.

I am hoping there won't be a third problem. The one unknown is what cemetery my mother wishes to be buried in after her passing. My final goal is to have her resting in the same cemetery as her parents. That remains the one unanswered question. Since one parent wishes to be cremated, and the other wishes to be buried after a viewing and funeral, it will only be a matter of time to find out how that situation is resolved. Expectations are that securing a burial plot will be an easy, uncomplicated task when the time comes.

PARKINSON'S VERSUS INDEPENDENCE

Much has been mentioned about Alzheimer's disease, but now it's time to discuss Parkinson's and its impact on my father and his behaviors. As you observe him in his daily routine of getting out medications, eating meals, changing channels on the television, you become aware of the slight tremors of the hands. While he watches the various channels, you also see he rubs his thumb and forefinger together in circular motions, or incessantly rubs them on the arm of his chair.

These movements are a visible indication of Parkinson's disease.

Independence is lost in the numerous attempts to work on the smallest of objects that once were fixed with ease. These days it is necessary for him to ask for help from a neighbor to change burned out light bulbs, or follow directions to assemble a grouping of shelves that hold a place in the living room for the telephone or remote controls of TVs, VCRs, and DVD players. Dad feels less useful since he has difficulty with movements involving small muscle coordination, as well as the loss of vision due to macular degeneration.

Writing and steadiness on the feet are also strong indicators of loss of muscle power. It is difficult for them to acknowledge the decline in age related processes. Once vibrant, alert, and contributors to society must now rely on others for care and reliable services. Remaining in their own home is the last piece of independence.

Lengthy strides that were visible during walks as a younger gentleman now give way to feet that shuffle along the sidewalk or flooring. A cane is used to assist with stability, but the balance is unsteady, so the pace has become extremely slow. Distances that used to require longer walks have now become drastically shortened due to lack of energy and stableness. Energetic behaviors give way to longer, more recurrent periods of resting in the personal lounge chair. Frequent naps become the routine custom. He is comfortable taking one day at a time since he considers this his retirement program.

Who's Calling, Please?

Phone calls create and maintain an important link across the miles. During Father's Day of 2008, I had the opportunity to make a long desired trip to New York to visit my oldest son and daughter-in-law. It had been several years since we had visited in person, so the anticipated trip was expected to be enjoyable for us to partake of some family bonding time again.

As the three of us drove north from New York City to the upper part of the state to visit my daughter-in-law's parents we chatted about life, the scenery, happenings in both families, and passed the time with engaging discussions that flowed endlessly. It was during the drive that we decided to contact my dad for a few moments of Father's Day banter about the day, as well as inform them about what was taking place on our end of the phone. Cell phones are a marvelous invention that allow for communication from anywhere in the USA. Since I was not the driver, I dialed the phone to contact the older parents/grandparents. The ringing of the phone was halted by my mother answering the call.

I began the phone greeting with, "Happy Father's Day!" I was anticipating her passing the phone to my dad. To my dismay, that was not the case.

The response on the other end of the phone line was, "Who's calling, please?"

For an instant I was stunned as the idea became clear that she did not recognize my voice, so I had to clarify that it was her daughter calling to wish Dad a Happy Father's Day! Eventually, she relinquished the phone to him, but not without reluctance on her part.

Not only was this a surprise, but now in 2009, we have experienced the fact that she has occasions when she does not recall her grandsons' names, names of each of their spouses, or any of their birthdays. That Father's Day episode was another notch on the Alzheimer's wall of missing information.

As we deal with the loss of memory, the daily phone calls contain moments of lucidity, as well as times of sheer panic when details from daily events can not be easily recalled. Patience is the word of the day when you have to fill in the missing information, or listen the recounting of the same details several times in the same conversation. This happens more and more frequently, not less often. Even with daily doses of medication to slow down the memory loss process, it's difficult to watch the perpetual memory failure happen to someone you love. Thinking appears to be temporarily shutting down. The elevator of thought processing seems to be stuck in between floors, or can seldom make its way to the top floor.

ANNIVERSARY PARTY

Sixty-five years of marriage is a mile stone for many older couples to achieve in this era. Marriages that were entered into by those individuals who are now octogenarians, or nonagenarians, were literally intended to last "till death do us part". To celebrate this event, my father had to resolve some internal conflicts. Those shall remain unknown to the rest of the world, but happened to cause a exceptionally difficult situation which eventually had a solution that appeased the natives.

Once there was a determination that the celebration would actually be held, he arranged on his own to solicit the services of a caterer, a restaurant, and the guest list. I finalized the guest list and all required addresses, and sent him the final list for his approval. All was going well. Invitations were ordered, printed, addressed, and mailed. Still the festivities were unknown to his long term spouse. So far, so good! Plans went along surprisingly without a hitch. We all know that even the best laid plans will have some minor difficulties, but once my mother had an inkling a party was in the planning stages, the kinks in the works began to unravel.

In his quest for planning, Dad had selected a restaurant from the phone book, called, and notified them that the number of celebrants would probably total 20 to 25.

Seemed like a nice crowd to expect, and an appropriate amount could be budgeted for expenses.

That's what he and I thought. Little did we realize that once my mother got wind of a celebration, she would throw a monkey wrench or two into the works. We had carefully and thoroughly planned the guest list. What we did not plan on was the RSVP notation on the invitations would be ignored by the invitees, and my mother, not I, would be notified as to who would be attending. This situation gummed up with works. If she didn't hear from those who were invited, she questioned each of us as to who all was on the guest list. We couldn't invite everyone on their list of 100 names provided by their Christmas card list, but we did ask those with whom they have the most contact. That answer was not sufficient, nor to her liking. The guest list continued to grow until the day prior to the festivities.

At this point, panic set in! Not with her. She was thrilled to be the center of attention. Panic and frustration set in with me! According to my new calculations the list was double the anticipated number. Of course, with the Alzheimer's, she wasn't completely certain who she had invited.

No amount of reasoning in the world could convince her that we didn't need the entire city to celebrate their wedding anniversary.

When it was all said and done, there were 42 attendees who came from several states, ala cart ordering from the menu, and everyone who attended had a wonderful time. They didn't seem to mind being served smaller pieces of cake.

It was amazing to see who arrived, since my father and I weren't really sure of the final guest list on the day of the party, but it all turned out well. The restaurant was very accommodating in adding more tables and chairs to the seating arrangement.

That will be the last big celebration. I have decided that even if they make it to the seventieth wedding anniversary, there will not be a shin-dig akin to that sixty-fifth anniversary. I am not sure I will have the wear-with-all to do it again.

To this day, when the party is discussed, my mother will comment on who was not invited.

That's one time I wish the Alzheimer's would kick in so she wouldn't recall who was or was not in attendance. Either way, according to her, it was my fault that someone was eliminated from the guest list! Maybe I should open up a complaint department of my own.

THE COMPLAINT IDIOSYNCRASY

In the time continuum of aging, it is interesting to note that personality traits become more pronounced as one grows older. Those folks who were happy with life as they progressed were also happier later in life. It's a glass half empty, glass half full type of thinking. Life is filled with optimists and pessimists. The complaint idiosyncrasy belongs to the pessimists who see the glass as half empty.

Lousy is one vocabulary word my mother uses excessively to describe the eggs she had for breakfast, the service from the restaurant where they last dined, or the maneuvering of the driver of the "Lift" who most recently took them to the doctor's office for a visit. It seldom matters who performed what service, it remained "lousy"" by her standards. Unfortunately, it also illustrates her feelings regarding the pie baked by their cleaning gal who attends to their needs every Friday.

My mother's perceptions of the glass half empty have become more observable as she progresses into her late 80s. This trend complicates the misnomer of having a "cleaning" lady attend to their home. Due to the clutter strewn throughout the entire house, it's a nightmare to consider cleaning any given area, yet my mother complains if the kitchen floor is not tended to on a weekly basis, nor is the task of dusting the furniture taken seriously, let alone the bathroom odors being attacked by an arsenal of cleaning products.

Not only are three to six hours a week insufficient for one to conscientiously put a serious dent in removal of clutter about the house, but for this person to adequately clean, as well as bake one pie each week for their consumption between Friday visits is beyond comprehension. In my estimation, three to six hours a week for a cleaning person to keep a head of the clutter, making a valiant attempt at cleaning, as well as maintain doing the weekly laundry piled in the basement, in addition to baking a pie is arduous.

Of course, the complaints are delivered after the three hours a day, two days a week, of doing the same tasks as were accomplished the previous week. Not only were the tasks not performed to satisfaction, but the hired cleaning girl made more of a mess baking the pie, than she had in the kitchen before she started. It's a no win situation with the complainers idiosyncrasies. The question I have to ask myself would be: "How much should I intervene?"

This is an elderly woman who would complain if you gave her a thousand dollar bill because she wanted one that wasn't wrinkled!

My guess regarding the complaint about the pie is: "It's made of lousy apples!"

To Move or Not To Move

During the past six years, one nagging question has crept in and out of the background of conversations. Should they move into an assisted living facility that had their own nursing staff, or possibly consider a retirement community for elderly who still maintained some independence? Many of their friends had taken the last choice and became citizens of a retirement community. There were various reasons or excuses for my parent's hesitation to leave their personal residence and move into a senior living building with various sized apartments that suited ones particular needs.

Discussions ensued regarding the possibility of making a choice between assisted living or retirement communities. Comparing and contrasting each after several visits gave more meaning to the ongoing conversations, but there were more excuses why they should not move than there were reasons why they should move from the quaint red brick house.

Debates concerned living space, and the tiny, cramped quarters presented in most of the assisted living facilities. Usually the apartments visited had one bedroom, a small kitchen, limited closet space, and an undersized bathroom. Going from a two bedroom, one bath home with a full basement and attic would definitely require elimination of many personal effects. This became excuse number one.

Once we ruled out the assisted living apartments, it was time to revert back to discussions which revolved around the retirement community services and the variety of apartments which they offered for graduated fees. These dwellings were much larger in comparison. Both types of facilities offered the availability of placement on a waiting list once a decision was made by the interested parties.

Finally, a selection was made on a cozy two bedroom, two bath apartment that also had a larger living room, and kitchen where meals could be easily created for two adults. The internal porch-like door was complete with a lamp that gently illuminated the entrance. Security checked each apartment by a specified time every morning. If the porch light had not been turned off, the occupants were looked in on as a precautionary measure. The ground floor apartments also provided access to a small cement patio area for the resident's personal enjoyment. It appeared that a selection between living facilities had been made, and the required monies were given for a deposit. Their names were placed appropriately on the waiting list. It seemed success was eminent. It would only be a matter of time before they would join a few of their long time friends and become residents of this facility nestled among colorful gardens and tall maple trees. It wouldn't be long before an apartment of their choice would be available for the anticipated move.

At this writing, it has been six years, and several dozen phone calls from the facility to alert the folks that an apartment is obtainable. Offers are made by the manager of the complex, discussed, and promptly declined. We now have serious discussions as to why the numerous openings have been passed over. The understanding for pending moves is that this elderly couple is free to decline one apartment in hopes that the next one will fit into the scheme of things.

Upon further inspection of the reasons provided, the discovery of the list of excuses become more and more apparent. One excuse given was it was too far to walk to the dining hall if they don't want to cook, but want to eat their meals in the centrally located dining room with other residents. Another excuse involved the location and placement of the organ that had to be moved from point A, the home, to point B, the apartment, and the lay out of the apartment itself.

The final excuse that brought all future conversations that surrounded the move to a screeching halt was the one regarding their porch swing. Approximately fifteen years ago a five foot long redwood swing, complete with its own stand and matching roof, was purchased for daily enjoyment outside during the summer months. Hours of companionship have been accumulated watching the neighbors walking their dogs, children riding on bikes, or traffic patterns as cars are seen driving up and down the street in front of their house. Towards the end of each summer they marvel at the nightly ritual of hearing and seeing the several flocks of Canadian geese flying in formation while passing overhead. Now the question to answer: "To move, or not to move?"

Although the ground floor apartments each have a patio for the location of the red wood swing, my father doesn't want to have to feel obligated to share the swing with other residents of the facility! What they feel are valid reasons have become excuses to remain in their home. Getting rid of the clutter and some possessions, moving the organ which is seldom played to another location, and not sharing the red wood swing have all become convenient excuses rather than legitimate reasons not to make the move to another residence.

FORTRESS OF PAPER

Boxes of old Christmas and birthday cards filled with good wishes, bills from the cable or electric company, church bulletins, bank statements, magazines, and numerous envelopes containing requests for donations all form a fortress around the recliner where my mother naps or watches television. Every envelope received is tossed in some sort of cardboard box, but prior to the discarding of each packet, not one escapes the display of a ragged, torn edge where the postage stamp used to be. A manila envelope contains the ripped pieces of envelopes that still have a cancelled stamp glued to the torn edge with its half inch border. These are collected for a friend who uses the stamps as donations to a support group in another country.

For elderly folks who do not venture out of the house very often, watching for the mailman who still walks his designated route becomes part of the morning ritual. The aged are aware of the mail truck that sits idly at the corner of the block as the mail carrier walks from house to house in the rain, sleet, or snow. Since they have followed his routine for the past fifteen years, they can predict how long it will take him to arrive at their home to deposit the handful of envelopes in their box at the foot of the cement stoop just outside the front door.

Once the daily mail has been deposited in their receptacle, either of them has the honor of retrieving the stack of bills and other notices, but usually the routine finds my father going out to get the mail and bringing it in the house so he can deposit the entire pile on the cushion of his wife's recliner. She will be the designee who opens all letters, reads them for content, then gives them a toss across the living room to Dad, who is also seated in his personal recliner for his perusal. Most mail is met with calm acceptance; however, those unsolicited requests for cash donations are met with the elder rage phenomenon.

As hard as I try, there is no persuasive technique known to man-kind that will convince this little old lady that her generosity has not gone unnoticed by those who seek her monetary support. Loss of memory causes her to display a misunderstanding of how these organizations acquired their name and address. It is difficult to convince my mother that due to the fact they donate on a regular basis to several selected associations, those societies in turn sell a list of names containing individuals who easily part with their cash. Companies, be they religious in nature, or just some organization that requests a donation for their cause, the ire exhibited is relentless and uncontrollable. These groups who solicit aid in funding their endeavors don't realize how much they contribute to the fortress of clutter that surrounds the recliner.

The most amazing part of this scenario is even with the shuffling of feet when walking, and the use of a cane for stability by both parents, neither of them has slipped and fallen on the papers which clutter the living room rug.

Fortress not-withstanding, most of the paper clutter belongs in one of the black trash bags for the upcoming Sunday midnight trash pick up!

LONGEVITY

All things considered, even with the macular degeneration and heart irregularities for both parents, and Alzheimer's that affect my mother, or the Parkinson's Disease that impairs my father's movements, they have managed to maintain their own home. The years of longevity have demonstrated their life existence far beyond other family members. Each of them is the lone survivor from each side of the family linage. They have even outlived their youngest son, as well as their youngest grandson.

Sixty-five years of wedded bliss surpasses the length of most marriages that are entered into in the past century. There are moments when they seem to resemble "Archie and Edith Bunker" in the way they interact; however, during other times life can be calm and uneventful. My father's passive resistance complements my mother's tumultuous rage. Her most organized area of expertise is seen in the finely balanced check book. During their life times, both were hard working, and dedicated to raising two children for whom they provided college educations.

They have seen a number of significant inventions including television, computers, cell phones, microwave ovens, air-conditioning, medical advances using penicillin, and witnessed space shuttles to the moon, just to name a few of the many improvements in the quality of human life.

Throughout the span of almost 100 years, they have remained true and constant to their faith. As strong believers who have a personal knowledge of a higher power, that conviction keeps them grounded.

I am not sure where the longevity comes from in this family, but I hope my sons are patient and understanding with me if I live to be a nonagenarian. Whatever the basis for the prolonged existence, I know no matter how you slice it, you can only eat one piece of pie at a time! Although apple, peach, pumpkin, raspberry, or cherry were among the most frequently consumed, there is one important bit of criteria: it must be an all time favorite piece of lemon meringue!

www.ingramcontent.com/pod-product-compliance
Lightning Source LLC
Chambersburg PA
CBHW020238290526
45784CB00003B/1024